The Ultimate Cookbook for Anti-Inflammatory Desserts

Delicious Ideas To Satisfy Your Sweet Tooth While Reducing the Inflammation in Your Body

By
Olga Jones

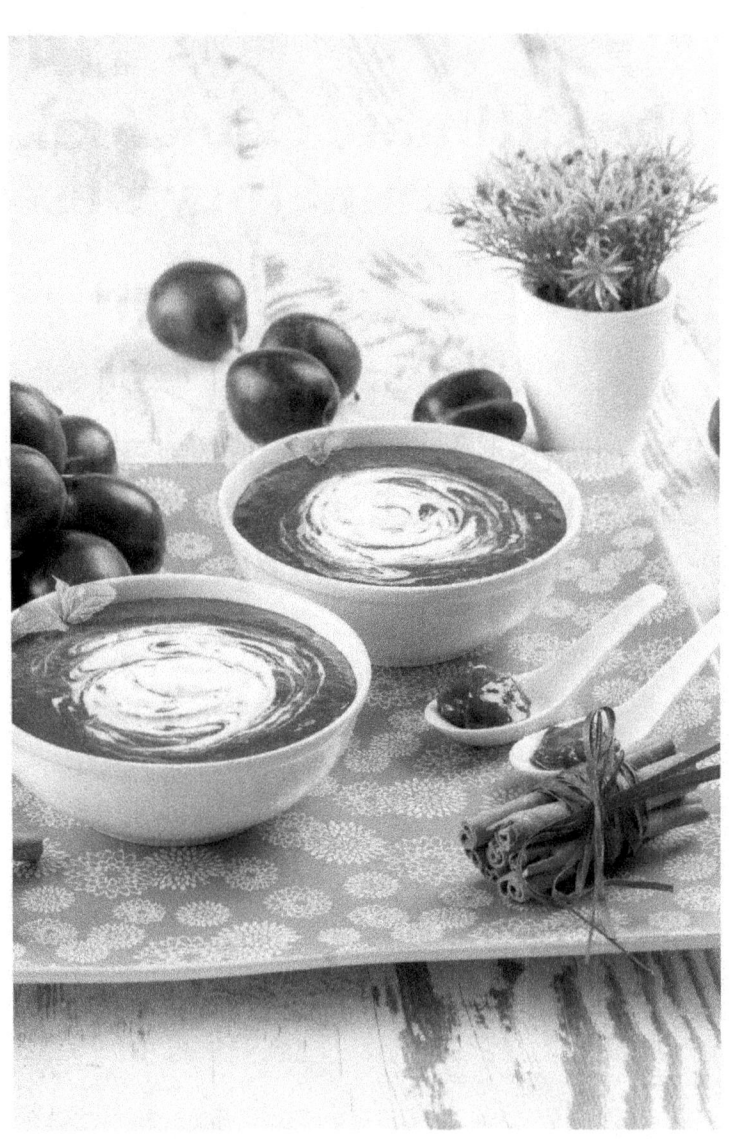

© Copyright 2021 by Olga Jones - All rights reserved. The following Book is reproduced below with the goal of providing information that is as accurate and reliable as possible. Regardless, purchasing this Book can be seen as consent to the fact that both the publisher and the author of this book are in no way experts on the topics discussed within and that any recommendations or suggestions that are made herein are for entertainment purposes only. Professionals should be consulted as needed prior to undertaking any of the action endorsed herein.

This declaration is deemed fair and valid by both the American Bar Association and the Committee of Publishers Association and is legally binding throughout the United States.

Furthermore, the transmission, duplication, or reproduction of any of the following work including specific information will be considered an illegal act irrespective of if it is done electronically or in print. This extends to creating a secondary or tertiary copy of the work or a recorded copy and is only allowed with the express written consent from the Publisher. All additional rights reserved.

The information in the following pages is broadly considered a truthful and accurate account of facts and as such, any inattention, use, or misuse of the information in question by the reader will render any resulting actions solely under their purview. There are no scenarios in which the publisher or the original author of this work can be in any fashion deemed liable for any hardship or damages that may befall them after undertaking information described herein.

Additionally, the information in the following pages is intended only for informational purposes and should thus be thought of as universal. As befitting its nature, it is presented without assurance regarding its prolonged validity or interim quality. Trademarks that are mentioned are done without written consent and can in no way be considered an endorsement from the trademark holder.

Table of Contents

INTRODUCTION 7
What is the Anti-Inflammatory Diet? 7
Vanilla Cakes 9
Watermelon Sorbet 11
No-Bake Strawberry Cheesecake 13
Blackberry & Apple Skillet Cake 15
Black Forest Pudding 18
Fried Pineapple Slices 19
Baked Apples 21
Rhubarb & Blueberry Granita 22
Pumpkin Ice-Cream 23
Pineapple & Banana Ice-Cream 25
Lemon Sorbet 26
Chocolate & Coffee Mousse 28
Chocolaty Chia Pudding 30
Apple Chia Pudding 31
Chocolate Custard 34
Strawberry Soufflé 36
Mango & Pineapple Crisp 38
Cherry Cobbler 40
No-Bake Lemony Cheesecake 42
Banana Mug Cake 44
Brown Rice Pudding 46
Pineapple Upside-Down Cake 48
Fudge Brownies 51
Lemony Tarts 53
Chocolaty Cherry Truffles 56

Almond Cookies	58
Apple Fritters	61
Avocado Chia Parfait	63
Avocado Chocolate Mousse	65
Banana Bars	67
Banana Cinnamon Cookies	68
Berry Ice Pops	71
Berry-Banana Yogurt	72
Blueberry Crisp	73
Blueberry Sour Cream Cake	75
Café-Style Fudge	77
Grams Choco Chia Cherry Cream	79
Chocolate Cherry Chia Pudding	80
Chocolate Chip Quinoa Granola Bars	82
Chocolate Fudge Bites	85
Cinnamon Apple Chips	86
Citrus Strawberry Granita	88
Coconut Butter Fudge	90
Coffee Cream	91
Cookie Dough Bites	93
Creamy Frozen Yogurt	94
Date Dough & Walnut Wafer	95
Fall-Time Custard	97
Flourless Sweet Potato Brownies	99
Fruit Cobbler	102
Glazed Banana	104
Green Tea Pudding	105
Hot Chocolate	106
Lemon Vegan Cake	108

INTRODUCTION

What is the Anti-Inflammatory Diet?

The anti-inflammatory diet is the best choice for your health if you have conditions that cause inflammation. Such conditions are asthma, chronic peptic ulcer, tuberculosis, rheumatoid arthritis, periodontitis, Crohn's disease, sinusitis, active hepatitis, etc. Along with medical treatment, proper nutrition is very important. An anti-inflammatory diet can help to reduce the pain from inflammation for a few notches. Such a diet isn't a panacea but a significant help in any treatment. Inflammation is a natural response of your body to infections, injuries, and illnesses. The classic symptoms of inflammation are redness, pain, heat, and swelling. Nevertheless, some diseases don't have any symptoms. Such illnesses are diabetes, heart disease, cancer, etc. That's why we should care about our health permanently and an anti-inflammatory diet is one of the ways for it.

Inflammation is your immune system's response to injury or unwanted microbes in your body. It is a natural process and vital part of your body's healing process. When inflammation becomes systemic and chronic, however, it becomes a problem, and measures need to be taken. This type of inflammation serves no purpose, and can cause a lot of harm to the body.

This book has a LOT of recipes, and not every recipe might work for you. For example, if you're allergic to dairy or gluten, the recipes containing those ingredients will cause more harm than good. However, substitutions are possible for all of these, so you will be fine following this book as long as you keep an eye on the ingredients and use a bit of creativity where you have to! Once you understand the fundamentals of the diet, you will be fully equipped to create your own recipes from scratch!This is the most important information that you should know before starting a diet. Any diet is not a magic remedy for all diseases; it is a support for the body during a difficult time of treatment. Start your new healthy life from one small step and you will see the huge results within half a year. You can be sure that your body will be thankful to you by giving you a fresh look and energy for new achievements.

Vanilla Cakes

TimeTo Prepare: ten minutes
Time to Cook: fifteen minutes
Yield: Servings 8

Ingredients: .
- 5 tsp. Baking soda .
- 5 tsp. Salt
- 1 cup Agave sweetener
- 1 cup Almond milk
- 1 tbsp. Apple cider vinegar
- 2 cup Whole wheat flour
- 2 tsp. Baking powder C.
- 5 cup warmed coconut oil
- tsp. Vanilla extract

Directions:
1. Ensure the oven is set to 350F.
2. Prepare two muffin pans (12 c) for use by greasing them.
3. Put in the apple cider vinegar into a measuring c that is big enough to hold minimum 2 c.
4. Put in the almond milk for a total of 1.5 c.

5. Allow the results to curdle roughly five minutes or until done.

6. Put together the salt, baking soda, baking powder, sugar, and flour together in a big container and whisk well.

7. Separately, mix the vanilla, coconut oil, and curdled almond in its container before combining the two bowls and blending well.

8. Put in the results to the muffin pans, dividing uniformly.

9. Put the muffin pans in your oven and allow them to cook for approximately fifteen minutes.

10. You will know if it's all already cooked when you can press down on the tops and spring back when pressed lightly.

11. Allow the cake pans to cool on a wire rack before removing the cakes for the best results.

Watermelon Sorbet

Time To Prepare: 5 Minutes

Time to Cook: fifteen Minutes

Yield: Servings 4

Ingredients:
- 1 Seedless Watermelon, cubed

Directions:

1. To start with, put the watermelon cubes in a baking sheet in a uniform layer.

2. Next, keep the sheet in the freezer for about two hours or until the watermelon is solid.

3. After this, move the frozen watermelon cubes in the high-speed blender and puree them until you get a smooth puree.

4. Next, pour the puree among the two loaf pans.

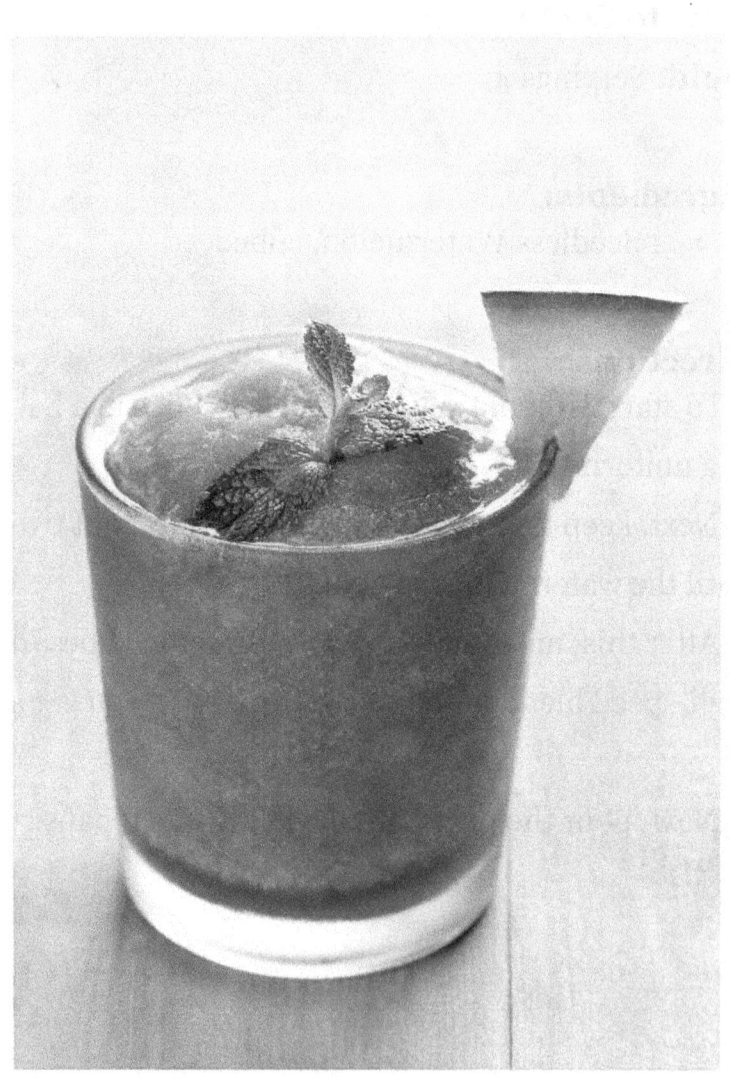

No-Bake Strawberry Cheesecake

Yield: 8 servings

Preparation Time: twenty minutes

Cooking Time: 5 minutes

Ingredients:
For Crust:
- 1 cup almonds
- 1 cup pecans
- 2 tablespoons unswee10ed coconut flakes
- 6 Medjool dates, pitted, soaked for 10 min and drained
- Pinch of salt

For Filling:
- 3 cups cashews, soaked and drained
- ¼ cup organic honey
- ¼ cup fresh lemon juice
- 1/3 cup coconut oil, melted
- 1 teaspoon organic vanilla flavor
- ¼ teaspoon salt
- 1 cup fresh strawberries, hulled and sliced

For Topping:
- 1/3 cup maple syrup
- 1/3 cup water
- Drop of vanilla flavor
- 5 cups fresh strawberries, hulled, sliced and divided

Directions:
1. Grease a 9-inch springform pan.
2. For the crust, in the small mixer, add almonds and pecans and pulse till finely grounded.
3. Add remaining all ingredients and pulse till smooth.
4. Transfer the crust mixture into the prepared pan, pressing gently downwards. Freeze to create completely.
5. In a large blender, add all filling ingredients and pulse till creamy and smooth.
6. Place the filling mixture over the crust evenly.
7. Freeze for at least a couple of hours or till set completely.
8. In a pan, add maple syrup, water, vanilla and 1 cup of strawberries on medium-low heat. 9. Bring to a gentle simmer. Simmer for around 4-5 minutes or till thickens.
10. Strain the sauce and allow it to go cool completely.
11. Top the chilled cheesecake with strawberry slices. Drizzle with sauce and serve.

Blackberry & Apple Skillet Cake

Yield: 4 servings

Preparation Time: 20 minutes

Cooking Time: 25 minutes

Ingredients:

For Filling:
- 2 tablespoons coconut oil
- 1 tablespoon coconut sugar
- 3 sweet apples, cored and cut into bite sized pieces
- ½ teaspoon ground cinnamon
- ¼ teaspoon ground cardamom
- 1/8 teaspoon ground cloves
- 1/8 teaspoon ground ginger
- 1 cup frozen blackberries

For Cake Mixture:
- ¾ cup ground almonds
- ½ teaspoon baking powder
- 2 tablespoons coconut sugar
- Pinch of salt
- ¼ cup full- Fat coconut milk
- 1 tablespoon coconut oil, melted
- 1 organic egg, bea10
- ½ teaspoon organic vanilla extract

Directions:
1. Preheat the oven to 40 degrees F.
2. In an ovenproof skillet, add butter and coconut sugar on high heat.
3. Cook, stirring for approximately 2-3 minutes.
4. Stir in apples and spices and cook, stirring approximately 5 minutes.
5. Remove from heat and stir in blackberries.
6. Meanwhile in a bowl, mix together ground almonds, baking powder, coconut sugar and salt.
7. In another bowl, add remaining ingredients and beat till well combined.
8. Add egg mixture into ground almond mixture and mix till well combined.
9. Place a combination over fruit mixture evenly.
10. Transfer the skillet into the oven.
11. Bake for approximately 15-20 min.
12. Serve warm.

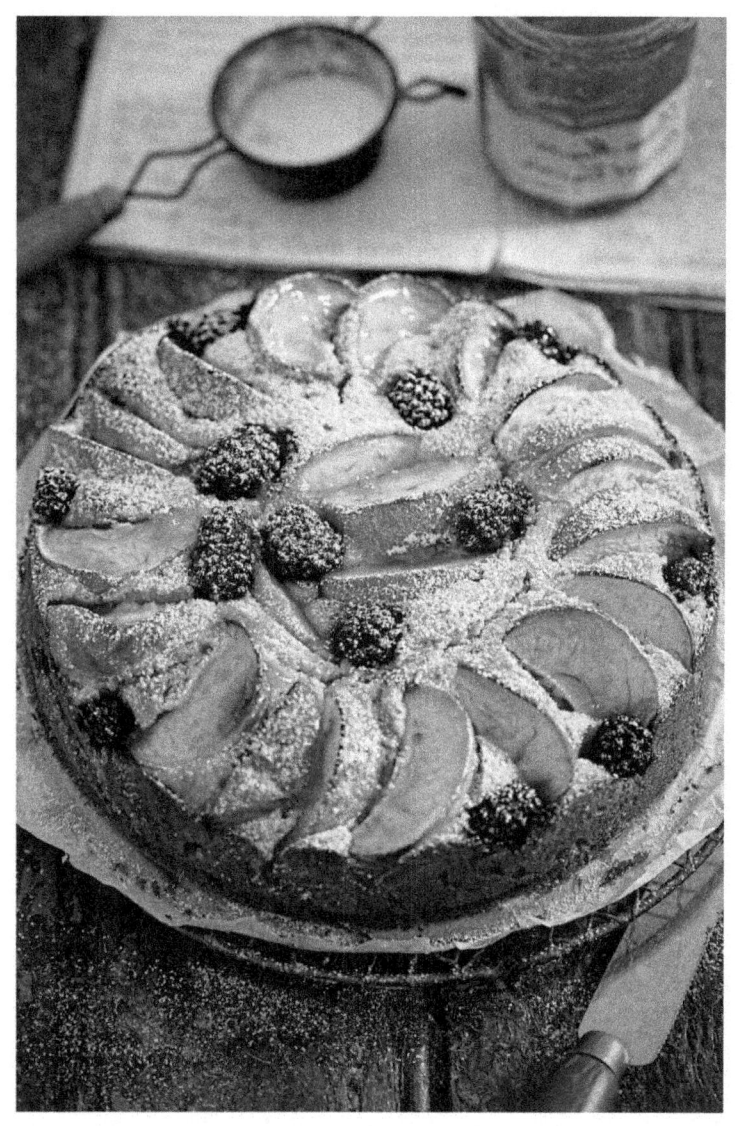

Black Forest Pudding

Yield: 2 servings

Preparation Time: 15 minutes

Cooking Time: 2 minutes

Ingredients:
- 1 teaspoon coconut cream
- 1 teaspoon coconut oil
- 3-4 squares 70% chocolate bars, chopped
- 1 cup coconut cream, whipped till thick and divided
- 2 cups fresh cherries, pitted and quartered
- 70% chocolate bars shaving, for garnishing
- Shredded coconut, for garnishing

Directions:

1. In a smaller pan, add 1 teaspoon coconut cream, coconut oil and chopped chocolate on low heat.
2. Cook, stirring continuously for about 2 minutes or till thick and glossy. Immediately, remove from heat.
3. In 2 serving glasses, divide chocolate sauce evenly.
4. Now, place ½ cup of cream over chocolate sauce in the glasses.
5. Divide cherries in glasses evenly.
6. Top with remaining coconut cream.
7. Garnish with chocolate shaving and shredded coconut.

Fried Pineapple Slices

Yield: 6-8 servings

Preparation Time: quarter-hour

Cooking Time: 6 minutes

Ingredients

- 1 fresh pineapple, peeled and cut into large slices
- ¼ cup coconut oil
- ¼ cup coconut palm sugar
- ¼ teaspoon ground cinnamon

Directions:

1. Heat a large surefire skillet on medium heat.
2. Stir in oil and sugar till coconut oil is very melted.
3. Add pineapple slices in batches and cook for approximately 1-2 minutes.
4. Carefully flip the side and cook for around 1 minute.
5. Cook for approximately 1 minute more.
6. Repeat with remaining slices.
7. Sprinkle with cinnamon and serve.

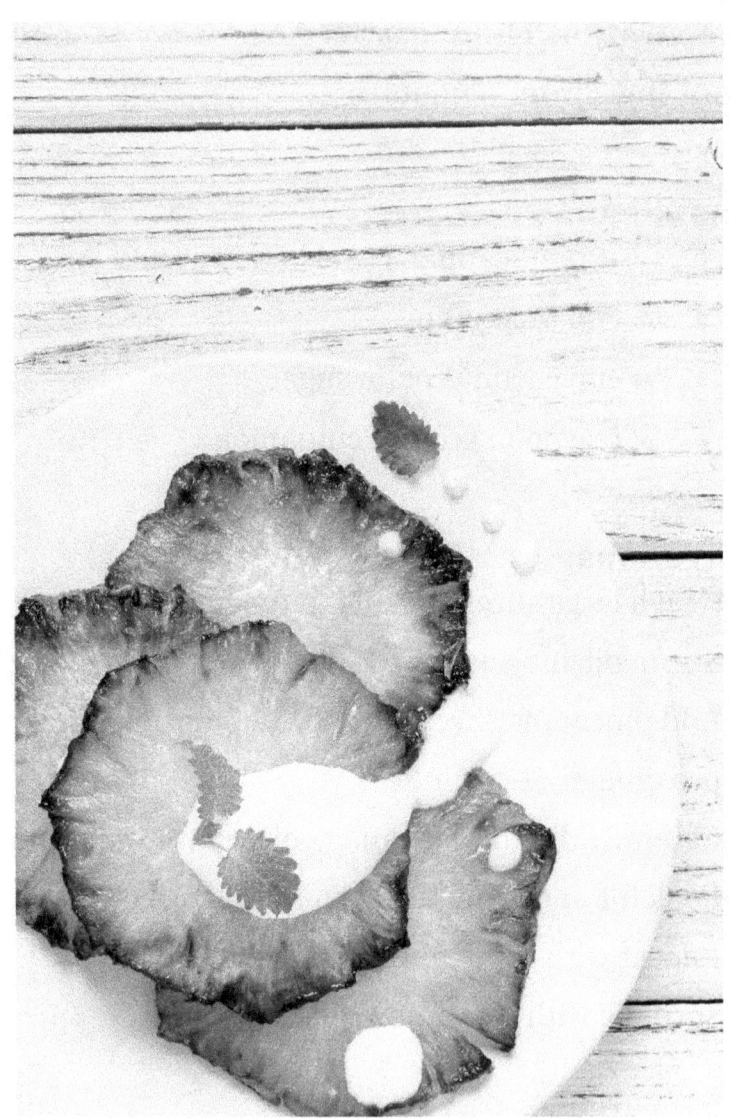

Baked Apples

Yield: 4 servings

Preparation Time: quarter-hour

Cooking Time: 18 minutes

Ingredients:

- 4 tart apples, cored
- ¼ cup coconut oil, softened
- 4 teaspoons ground cinnamon
- 1/8 teaspoon ground ginger
- 1/8 teaspoon ground nutmeg

Directions:

1. Preheat the oven to 350 degrees F.
2. Fill each apple with 1 tablespoon of coconut oil.
3. Sprinkle with spices evenly.
4. Arrange the apples onto a baking sheet.
5. Bake for around 12-18 minutes.

Rhubarb & Blueberry Granita

Yield: 8 servings

Preparation Time: 15 minutes

Cooking Time: 10 min

Ingredients:
- 1 cup fresh blueberries
- 3cups rhubarb, sliced
- ½ cup raw honey
- 2½ cups water
- Fresh mint leaves, for garnishing

Directions:

1. In a pan, add all ingredients on medium heat.
2. Cook, stirring occasionally for around 10 minutes.
3. Strain the mix through a strainer by pressing a combination.
4. Discard the pulp of fruit.
5. Transfer the strained mixture right into a 13x9-inch glass baking dish.
6. Freeze for around 20-a half-hour.
7. Remove from the freezer and with a fork scrap the mix.
8. Cover and freeze for approximately 60 minutes, scraping after every half an hour.

Pumpkin Ice-Cream

Yield: 6-8 servings

Preparation Time: quarter-hour

Ingredients:

- 1 (15-ounce) can pumpkin puree
- ½ cup dates, pitted and chopped
- 2 (14-ounce) cans coconut milk
- ½ teaspoon vanilla extract
- 1½ teaspoons pumpkin pie spice
- ½ teaspoon ground cinnamon
- Pinch of salt

Directions:

1. In an increased speed blender, add all ingredients and pulse till smooth.
2. Transfer into an airtight container and freeze for approximately 1-couple of hours.
3. Now, transfer into an ice-cream maker and process based on the manufacturer's directions.
4. Return the ice-cream into an airtight container and freeze for approximately 1-couple of hours.

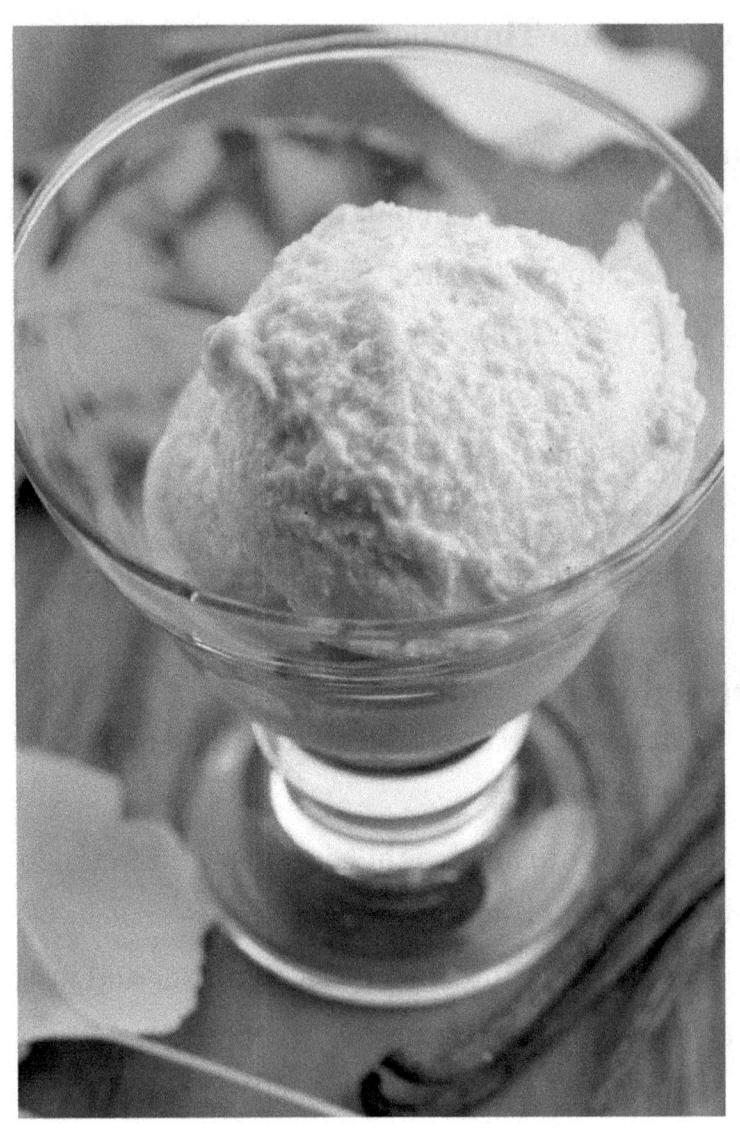

Pineapple & Banana Ice-Cream

Yield: 6 servings

Preparation Time: 15 minutes

Cooking Time: 20 min

Ingredients:
- 1(14-ounce) can coconut milk
- 1 cup frozen pineapple chunks, thawed
- 4 cups frozen banana slices, thawed
- 2 tablespoons fresh lime juice
- Pinch of salt

Directions:

1. Line a glass baking dish with plastic wrap.

2. In a higher speed blender, add all ingredients and pulse till smooth.

3. Transfer the amalgamation into the prepared baking dish evenly.

4. Freeze approximately 35-40 minutes.

Lemon Sorbet

Yield: 2 servings

Preparation Time: 10 minutes

Ingredients:
- 2 tablespoons fresh lemon zest, grated
- ½ cup raw honey
- 2 cups water
- 1½ cups freshly squeezed lemon juice

Directions:
1. Freeze ice-cream maker tub for about one day prior to sorbet.
2. In a pan, add all ingredients except fresh lemon juice on medium heat.
3. Simmer, stirring for approximately 1 minute or till sugar dissolves.
4. Remove from heat and stir in fresh lemon juice.
5. Transfer into an airtight container.
6. Refrigerate approximately 2 hours.
7. Now, transfer into an ice-cream maker and process according to manufacturer's directions.
8. While motor is running, add 1 tablespoon of oil.
9. Return the ice-cream into an airtight container and freeze approximately 120 minutes.

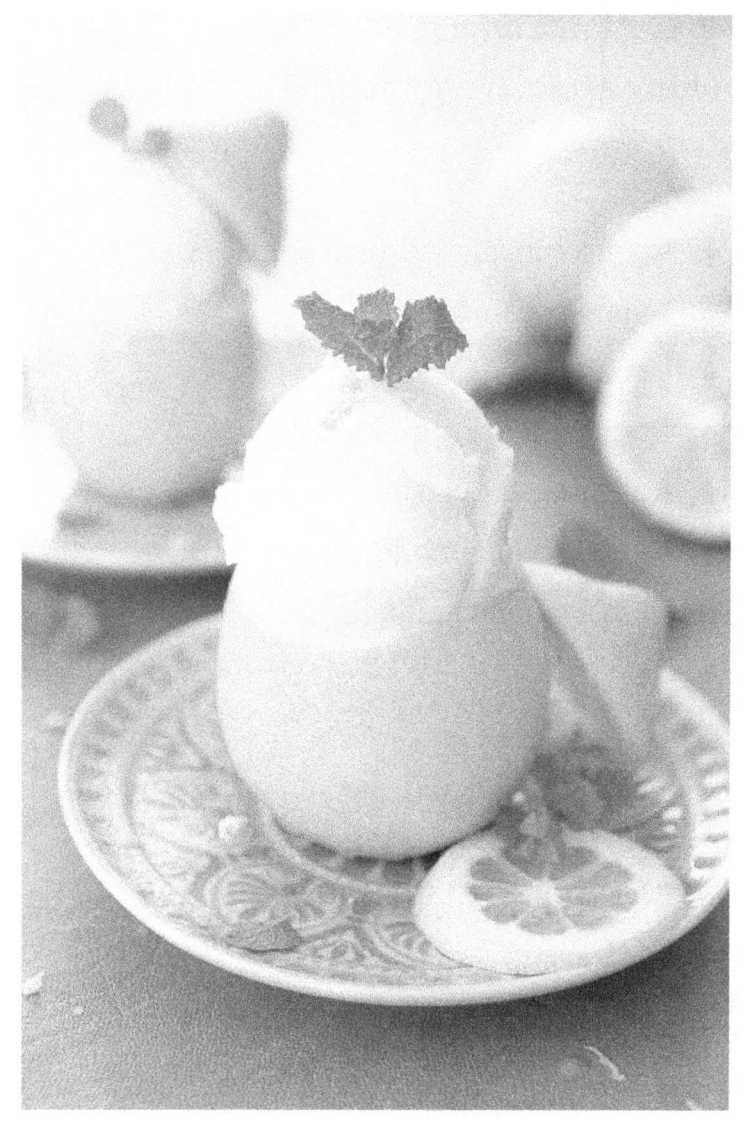

Chocolate & Coffee Mousse

Yield: 4 servings

Preparation Time: quarter-hour

Cooking Time: twenty minutes

Ingredients:
- ¼ cup chocolate brown chips
- ½ cup coconut milk
- ¼ cup boiling water
- 1 tablespoon ground coffees
- Raw honey, to taste
- ¼ teaspoon almond extract
- 1 tablespoon vanilla flavor

Directions:

1. In a nonstick pan, add chocolate chips on medium-low heat.
2. Cook, stirring continuously for around 2-3 minutes or till chocolate chips are melted.
3. Add coconut milk and beat till well combined.
4. Cook, stirring continuously for around 1-2 minutes.
5. Meanwhile in a small bowl, mix together hot water and coffee beans.

6. In a sizable bowl, add chocolate mixture, coffee mixture, honey and both extracts and mix till well combined.
7. Transfer the mousse in 4 serving glasses.
8. Refrigerate to relax for approximately 2-3 hours.

Chocolaty Chia Pudding

Yield: 4 servings

Preparation Time: 10 min

Ingredients:
- 6-9 dates, pitted and chopped
- 1½ cups unsweetened almond milk
- 1/3 cup chia seeds
- ¼ cup unsweetened cocoa powder
- ½ teaspoon ground cinnamon
- Salt, to taste
- ½ teaspoon vanilla flavor

Directions:
1. In a mixer, add all ingredients and pulse till smooth.
2. Transfer the mixture into serving bowls.
3. Refrigerate to chill completely before serving.

Apple Chia Pudding

Yield: 1 serving

Preparation Time: fifteen minutes

Cooking Time: 20 minutes

Ingredients:
- ½ cup unsweetened almond milk
- 2 tablespoons chia seeds
- ½ teaspoon ground cinnamon, divided
- 1/8 teaspoon vanilla extract
- 1 apple, cored and chopped finely
- ½ teaspoon raw honey
- 1½ teaspoons water
- 2 tablespoons golden raisins

Directions:

1. In a bowl, mix together almond milk, chia seeds, ¼ teaspoon of cinnamon and vanilla flavoring.
2. Refrigerate for around 1-120 minutes.
3. In a microwave safe bowl, mix together apple, honey, water and remaining cinnamon and microwave on high for around 1-2 minutes, stirring once.
4. Remove from microwave and stir in raisins.
5. Add 50 % of apple mixture in chia seeds mixture and stir to blend.

6. Refrigerate before serving.

7. Top with remaining apple mixture and serve.

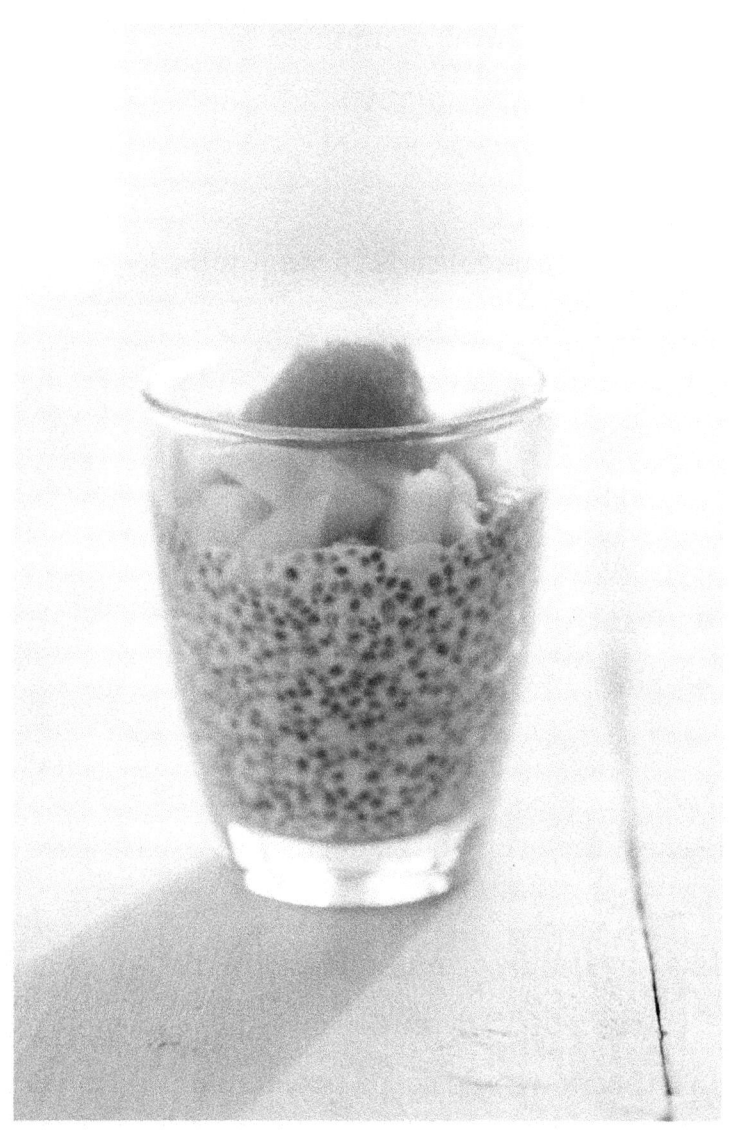

Chocolate Custard

Yield: 4-8 servings

Preparation Time: 15 minutes

Cooking Time: 35 minutes

Ingredients:
- 1½ (14-ounce) cans coconut milk
- 5 large organic eggs
- ½ cup raw honey
- 1 tablespoon vanilla flavor
- 3 tablespoons powdered cocoa
- 2 tablespoons trouble
- Pinch of ground cinnamon
- Pinch of ground nutmeg

Directions:
1. Preheat the oven to 325 degrees F. Grease a casserole dish.
2. In a bowl, add coconut milk, eggs and honey and beat till well combined.
3. In a tiny bowl, add cocoa powder and warm water and mix till a paste forms.
4. Add chocolate paste in eggs mixture and stir to blend.
5. Transfer the mixture into prepared casserole dish evenly.

6. Sprinkle with cinnamon and nutmeg.

7. Arrange the casserole dish in a large baking dish.

8. Pour the boiling water in baking dish about midway of the casserole dish.

9. Bake for about 35 minutes or till a toothpick inserted inside the center comes out clean.

Strawberry Soufflé

Yield: 6 servings

Preparation Time: quarter-hour

Cooking Time: 12 minutes

Ingredients:
- 18-ounce fresh strawberries, hulled
- 1/3 cup raw honey, divided
- 5 organic egg whites, divided
- 4 teaspoons fresh lemon juice

Directions:
1. Preheat the oven to 350 degrees F.
2. In a blender, add strawberries and pulse till a puree forms.
3. Through a strainer, strain the seeds.
4. In a bowl, add strawberry puree, 3 tablespoons of honey, 2 egg whites and lemon juice and pulse till frothy and light-weight.
5. In another bowl, add remaining egg whites and beat till frothy.
6. While beating gradually, add remaining honey and beat till stiff peaks form.
7. Gently, fold the egg whites into strawberry mixture.
8. Transfer the amalgamation into 6 large ramekins evenly.

9. Arrange the ramekins in a baking sheet.

10. Bake for approximately 10-12 minutes.

Mango & Pineapple Crisp

Yield: 6 servings

Preparation Time: quarter-hour

Cooking Time: fifteen minutes

Ingredients:
For Filling:
- 2 tablespoons coconut oil
- 2 tablespoons coconut sugar
- 1 large mango, peeled, pitted and cut into chunks
- 1 large pineapple, peeled and cut into chunks
- 1/8 teaspoon ground cinnamon
- 1/8 teaspoon ground ginger

For Topping:
- ¾ cup almonds
- 1/3 cup coconut, shredded
- ½ teaspoon ground allspice
- ½ teaspoon ground cinnamon
- ½ teaspoon ground ginger

Directions:
1. Preheat the oven to 375 degrees F.
2. For filling in the pan, melt coconut oil on medium-low heat.

3. Add coconut sugar and cook, stirring approximately 1-2 minutes.

4. Stir in remaining ingredients and cook for approximately 5 minutes.

5. Remove from heat and transfer the mixture in a baking dish.

6. Meanwhile for topping in a blender, add all ingredients and pulse till a coarse meal forms. 7. Place the topping over filling evenly.

8. Bake for approximately fifteen minutes or top becomes golden brown.

Cherry Cobbler

Yield: 4 servings

Preparation Time: fifteen minutes

Cooking Time: 25 minutes

Ingredients:
- 2 cups fresh cherries, pitted
- ¼ cup plus 1 tablespoon coconut palm sugar, divided
- ¼ cup pecans, chopped
- ¼ cup unsweetened coconut, shredded
- ¼ cup coconut flour
- 1 tablespoon arrowroot flour
- ½ teaspoon ground cinnamon
- Pinch of salt

Directions:
1. Preheat the oven to 375 degrees F.
2. In a 7x5-inch baking dish, position the cherries.
3. Place ¼ cup of coconut sugar over cherries evenly.
4. In a bowl, add 1 tablespoon of coconut sugar and remaining ingredients.
5. Spread pecan mixture over cherries evenly.
6. Bake for around 20-25 minutes.

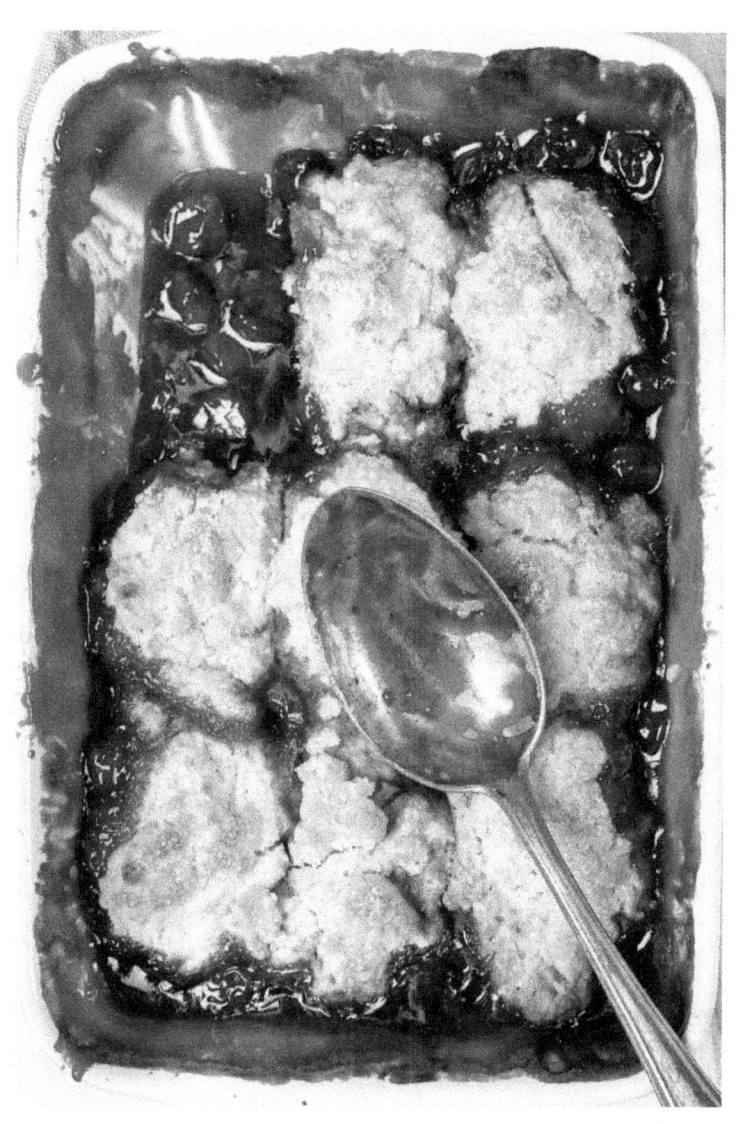

No-Bake Lemony Cheesecake

Yield: 12 servings

Preparation Time: twenty minutes

Ingredients:
For Crust:
- 1 cup dates, pitted and chopped
- 1 cup raw almonds
- 2-3 tablespoons unsweetened coconut, shredded

For Filling:
- 3½ cups cashews, soaked for overnight
- ½ cup coconut oil, melted
- 2 tablespoons fresh lemon rind, grated finely
- ¾ cup fresh lemon juice
- ¾ cup raw honey
- 10 drops liquid stevia
- 1 teaspoon vanilla flavoring
- Salt, to taste
- 1 lemon, sliced thinly

Directions:
1. In a blender, add dates, almonds and coconut and pulse till mixture just starts to blend.
2. Transfer the amalgamation in a greased springform pan.

3. With the back of the spatula, smooth the top of the crust.

4. In a food processor, add cashews and oil and pulse till well combined.

5. Add remaining ingredients except lemon slices and pulse till creamy and smooth.

6. Place the mixture over the crust evenly.

7. With the back of the spatula, smooth the surface of filling.

8. Refrigerate for about 60 minutes.

Banana Mug Cake

Yield: 1 serving

Preparation Time: 10 minutes

Cooking Time: 2 minutes

Ingredients:
- 1 banana, peeled a mashed
- 3 tablespoons almond meal
- ½ teaspoon baking powder
- 1 tablespoon coconut sugar
- ½ teaspoon ground cinnamon
- Pinch of ground ginger
- Pinch of salt
- 1 tablespoon coconut oil, softened
- ½ teaspoon vanilla extract

Directions:

1. In a bowl, add all ingredients and mix till well combined.
2. Transfer the amalgamation right into a microwave safe mug.
3. Microwave on high for about 2 minutes.

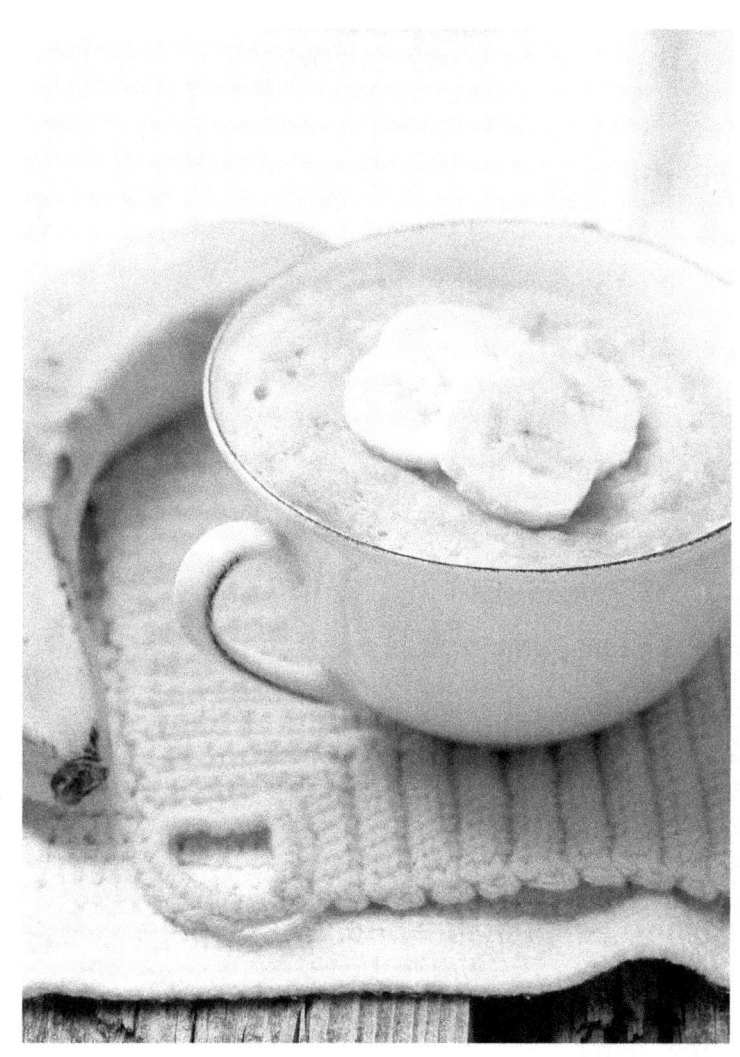

Brown Rice Pudding

Yield: 6-8 servings

Preparation Time: quarter-hour

Cooking Time: twenty minutes

Ingredients:
- 2 cups cooked brown rice
- 2 cups coconut milk
- 2 large organic eggs
- ¼ cup raw honey
- 1 teaspoon fresh lemon zest, grated finely
- 1 teaspoon ground cinnamon
- ½ teaspoon ground ginger
- ½ teaspoon ground cardamom
- ¼ teaspoon fresh ginger, grated finely
- 1 banana, peeled and sliced
- ¼ cup almond flakes

Directions:

1. Preheat the oven to 390 degrees F. Grease a baking dish.

2. Place cooked rice inside the bottom of the prepared baking dish evenly.

3. In a big bowl, add coconut milk, eggs, honey, lemon zest and spices and beat till well combined.

4. Place the egg mixture over rice evenly and top with banana slices and almonds.

5. Bake for around 20 minutes.

Pineapple Upside-Down Cake

Yield: 6 servings

Preparation Time: 15 minutes

Cooking Time: 50 minutes

Ingredients:

- 5 tablespoons raw honey, divided
- 2 (½-inch thick) fresh pineapple slices
- 15 fresh sweet cherries
- 1 cup almond flour
- 12 teaspoon baking powder
- 2 organic eggs
- 3 tablespoons coconut oil, melted
- 1 teaspoon vanilla extract
- Fresh cherries, for garnishing

Directions:

1. Preheat the oven to 350 degrees F.
2. In an 8-inch round cake pan, place about 1½ tablespoons of honey evenly.
3. Arrange the pineapple slices and 15 cherries over honey within your desired pattern.
4. Bake for approximately 15 minutes.
5. 1n a bowl, mix together almond flour and baking powder.

6. In another bowl, add eggs and remaining honey and beat till creamy.

7. Add coconut oil and vanilla extract and beat till well combined.

8. Add flour mixture into egg mixture and mix till well combined.

9. Remove the wedding cake pan from the oven.

10. Place the flour mixture over pineapple and cherries evenly.

11. Bake for approximately 35 minutes.

12. Remove from the oven and set aside to chill for approximately 10 min.

13. Carefully invert the dessert onto a serving plate.

14. Garnish with cherries and serve.

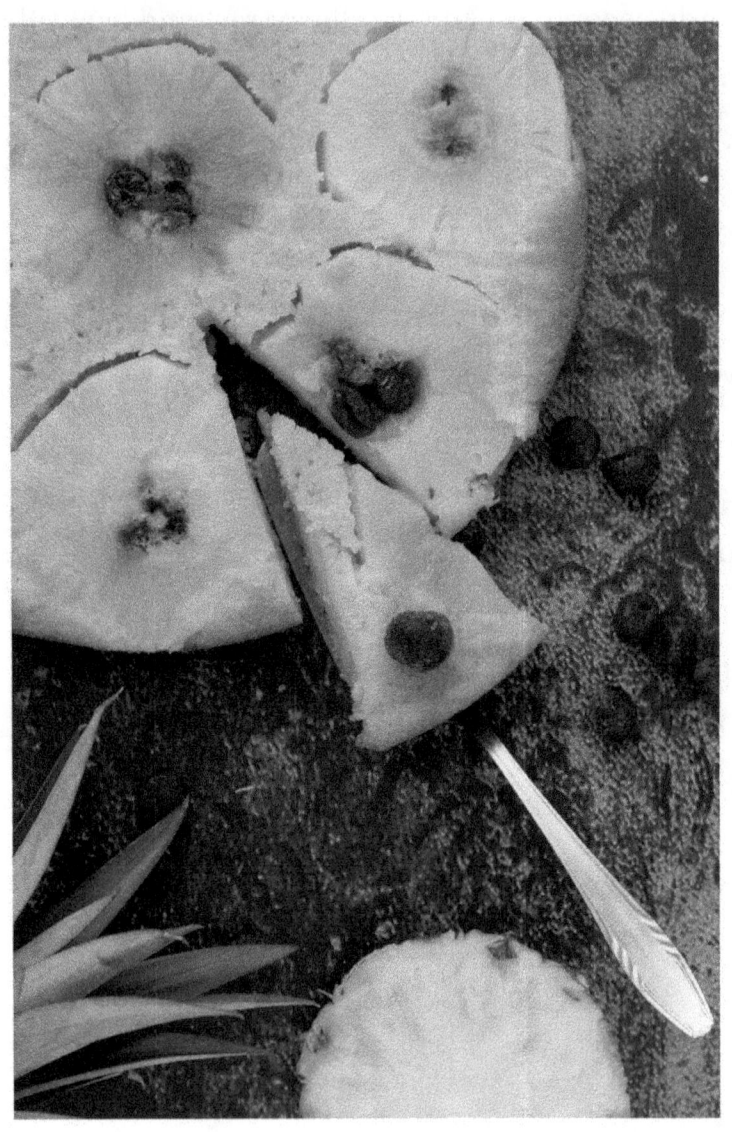

Fudge Brownies

Yield: 9 servings

Preparation Time: 15 minutes

Cooking Time: 26 minutes

Ingredients:
- 2-ounce unsweetened dark chocolate, chopped roughly
- ½ cup cocoa powder
- ½ cup coconut oil, melted
- ¾ cup raw honey
- 2 organic eggs
- 1 teaspoon vanilla extract
- ¼ cup coconut flour
- Salt, to taste

Directions:
1. Preheat the oven to 350 degrees F. Line a 9x9-inch baking dish using a greased parchment paper.
2. In a medium nonstick pan, mix together the chocolate, powdered cocoa and coconut oil on medium heat.
3. Cook, beating continuously approximately 2-3 minutes or till the amalgamation becomes smooth.
4. Remove from heat and immediately, stir in honey.

5. Add the eggs and vanilla flavoring and beat till well combined.

6. Transfer the amalgamation into the prepared baking dish evenly.

7. With the back of the spatula, smooth the very best surface.

8. Bake for around 20-23 minutes or till a toothpick inserted inside the center happens clean. 9. Remove from the oven and put it aside to cool completely.

10. After cooling, cut into desired size squares and serve.

Lemony Tarts

Yield: 4 servings

Preparation Time: 15 minutes

Cooking Time: quarter-hour

Ingredients:
For Crust:

- 1 cup almond meal
- 4 teaspoon dates, pitted
- 3 tablespoons fresh lemon juice

For Filling:

- 2 teaspoons fresh lemon zest, grated finely
- 1/3 cup fresh lemon juice
- 1 tablespoon raw honey
- 2 organic eggs, beaten

Directions:
1. Preheat the oven to 350 degrees F. Line 4 muffin cups with paper liners.
2. For the crust, inside a food processor, add all ingredients and pulse till well combined.
3. Place the amalgamation into prepared muffin cups and press firmly inside the bottom or more sides.

4. Bake for approximately 10-12 minutes.

5. Meanwhile in a pan, mix together all the filling ingredients except egg on low heat.

6. Simmer for about 2 minutes.

7. Slowly, add the eggs, beating continuously till well combined.

8. Remove from heat and put it aside to cool for around 5 minutes.

9. Place the filling inside the shells and refrigerate to cool.

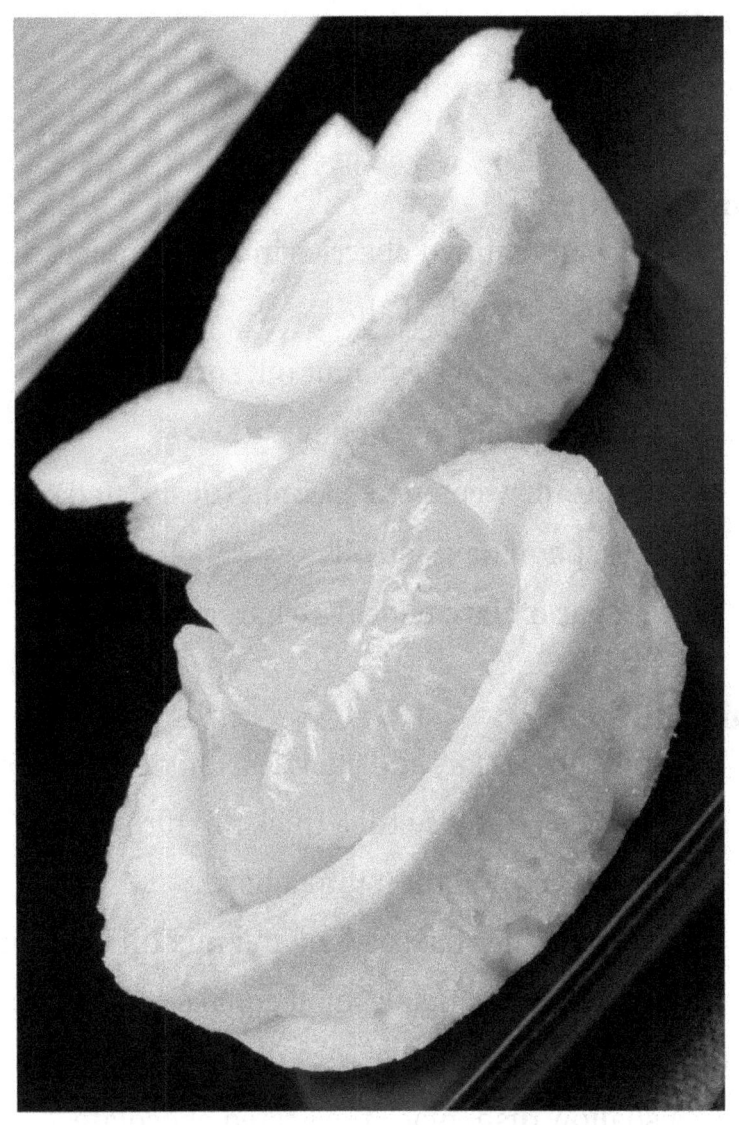

Chocolaty Cherry Truffles

Yield: 10-11 serving

Preparation Time: twenty minutes

Ingredients:
- 2½ cups canned cherries in natural juice, drained
- 2 cups almond meal
- 1½ tablespoons coconut oil, sof10ed
- 2 tablespoons raw honey
- 3 cups unsweetened coconut (desiccated)
- 1 teaspoon flaxseed oil
- 2/3 bar of dark chocolate bar, grated finely

Directions:
1. In a food processor, add cherries, almond meal, coconut oil and honey and pulse till a thick mixture forms.
2. Transfer a combination into a bowl.
3. Add coconut and flaxseed oil and mix till well combined.
4. With your hands, make small equal sized balls through the mixture.
5. In a shallow dish, place the grated chocolate.
6. Roll the balls in chocolate evenly.
7. Arrange the balls onto a parchment paper lined baking sheet.

8. With a plastic wrap, cover the baking sheet and refrigerate for about 2-3 hours.

Almond Cookies

Time To Prepare: fifteen min

Time to Cook: fifteen min

Yield: Servings 12

Ingredients:
- ½ tsp honey
- ½ tsp vanilla
- 1.7oz / 50g coconut butter
- 14oz / 400g non-wheat flour
- 1tsp baking powder
- 1tsp baking soda
- 3.5oz / 100g tahini
- Salt

Directions:

1. Combine the flour, soda, salt, baking powder together.

2. Mix tahini and coconut butter together and put in 2 tbsp. water in the same container.

3. Put in honey, vanilla to the tahini mixture and blend it well with a mixer.

4. Preheat the oven (180C/356F) and place a baking sheet on it.

5. Put in 24 tablespoons of the mixture onto the baking sheet and allow it to bake in your oven for 11-fifteen minutes.

6. Allow it to get cold a little bit before you serve.

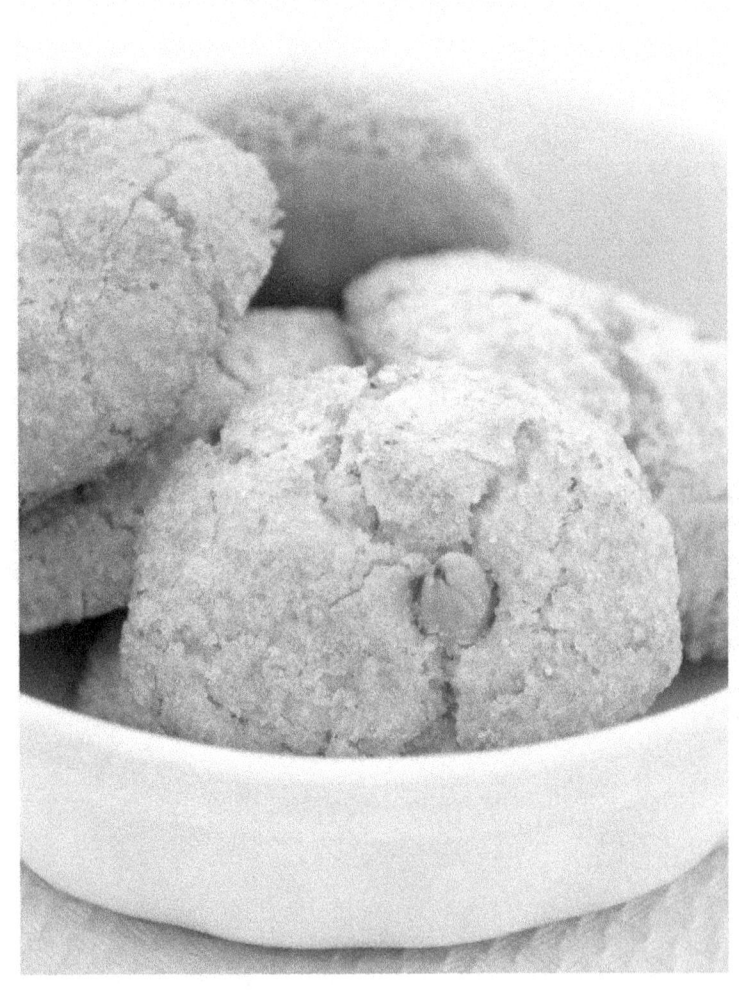

Apple Fritters

Time To Prepare: fifteen minutes
Time to Cook: ten minutes
Yield: Servings 4

Ingredients:

- ½ cup cashew milk
- 1 apple, cored, peeled, and chopped
- 1 cup all-purpose flour
- 1 egg
- 1½ teaspoons of baking powder
- 2 tablespoons of stevia sugar

Directions:

1. Preheat the air fryer to 175 degrees C or 350 degrees F.
2. Place parchment paper at the bottom of your fryer.
3. Line with cooking spray.
4. Mix together ¼ cup sugar, flour, baking powder, egg, milk, and salt in a container.
5. Mix well by stirring.
6. Drizzle 2 tablespoons of sugar on the apples. Coat well.
7. Mix the apples into your flour mixture.
8. Use a cookie scoop and drop the fritters with it to the air fryer basket's bottom.

9. Now air fry for five minutes.

10. Flip the fritters once and fry for another three minutes.

11. They must be golden.

Avocado Chia Parfait

Time ToPrepare: five minutes

Time to Cook: twenty minutes

Yield: Servings 2

Ingredients:
- ⅛ teaspoon nutmeg powder
- ½ teaspoon cinnamon powder
- ¾ teaspoon cinnamon powder
- 1 banana, mashed
- 1 tablespoon cashew nuts, chopped
- 1¼ cups almond milk
- 2 avocados, diced
- 2 tablespoons chia seeds
- 2 tablespoons pumpkin seeds
- Pinch of sea salt

Directions:
1. In a container, mix almond milk, banana, nutmeg powder, cinnamon powder, and pumpkin seeds.
2. Mix until well blended.
3. Chill in your refrigerator.
4. In the meantime, put the deep cooking pan on moderate heat.

5. Mix avocados, nutmeg powder, cinnamon powder, and salt.

6. Bring to its boiling point.

7. Allow simmering for about twenty minutes.

8. Remove the heat.

9. Mash half of the jam using a wooden spoon. Allow to cool. Set aside.

10. Ladle 2 tablespoons of parfait base and apple jam into parfait glasses.

11. Decorate using cashew nuts and serve

Avocado Chocolate Mousse

Time To Prepare: ten minutes

Time to Cook: 0 minute

Yield: Servings 9

Ingredients:
- ¼ cup espresso beans, ground
- ¼ cup of cocoa powder
- ½ teaspoon salt
- 1 bar dark chocolate
- 1 teaspoon vanilla extract
- 1/8 cup almond milk, unsweetened
- 2 tablespoons raw honey
- 3 ripe avocado, pitted and flesh scooped out
- 6 ounces plain
- Greek yogurt

Directions:
1. Put all ingredients in a food processor Pulse until the desired smoothness is achieved.
2. Best enjoyed chilled.

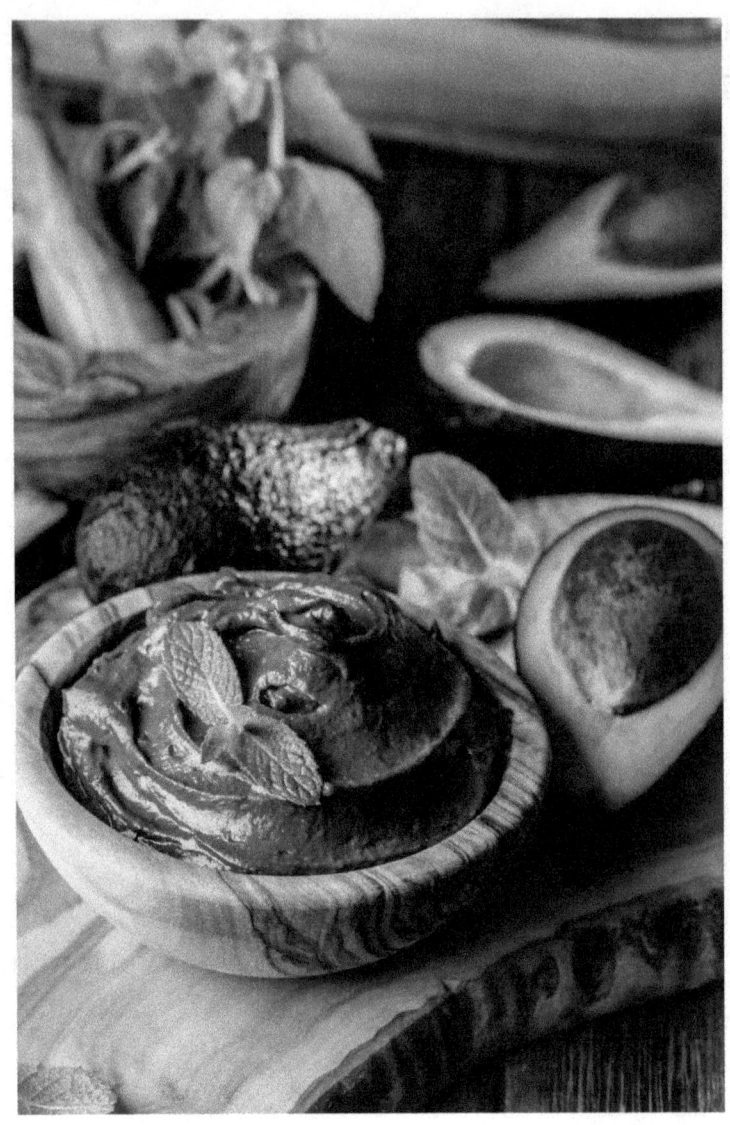

Banana Bars

Time To Prepare: ten minutes
Time to Cook: 60 minutes
Yield: Servings 4

Ingredients:
- ½ Cup Coconut Milk
- ½ Cup Melted Butter
- 1 Cup Chocolate Chips
- 1 Tsp. Baking Soda
- 1 Tsp. Pure Vanilla Extract
- 1/4 Tbsp. Cinnamon
- 2 Cup Brown Sugar
- 2 Cup Whole Wheat Flour
- 2 Eggs
- 5 Cup Ripe Mashed Banana
- Salt

Direction:
1. Preheat your oven to 170C.
2. Mix all together the ingredients to make the batter.
3. Put the batter in a wide tray and bake for about twenty minutes at 170C.
4. Serve with liquid chocolate or fruits.

Banana Cinnamon Cookies

Time To Prepare: five minutes

Time to Cook: ten minutes

Yield: Servings 2

Ingredients:
- 2 ripe bananas, peeled
- ¼ cup almond milk, unsweetened
- 4 pitted dates
- 1 tablespoon cinnamon
- 1 teaspoon vanilla
- 1 ½ teaspoon lemon juice
- 3 tablespoons dried and chopped cranberries
- 1 teaspoon baking powder
- 2 tablespoons dried and chopped raisins
- 2/3 cup applesauce, unsweetened
- 2/3 cup coconut flour

Directions:
1. Preheat your oven to 350 degrees F.
2. Use a food processor to mix almond milk, applesauce, dates, and bananas.
3. Blend until you achieve a smooth consistency.

4. Put in coconut flour, baking powder, cinnamon, vanilla, and lemon juice.

5. Blend for a minute.

6. Fold in cranberries and raisins.

7. Pour a baking sheet with the cookie dough.

8. Put inside the oven for about twenty minutes.

9. Let sit for five minutes and allow it to harden and serve.

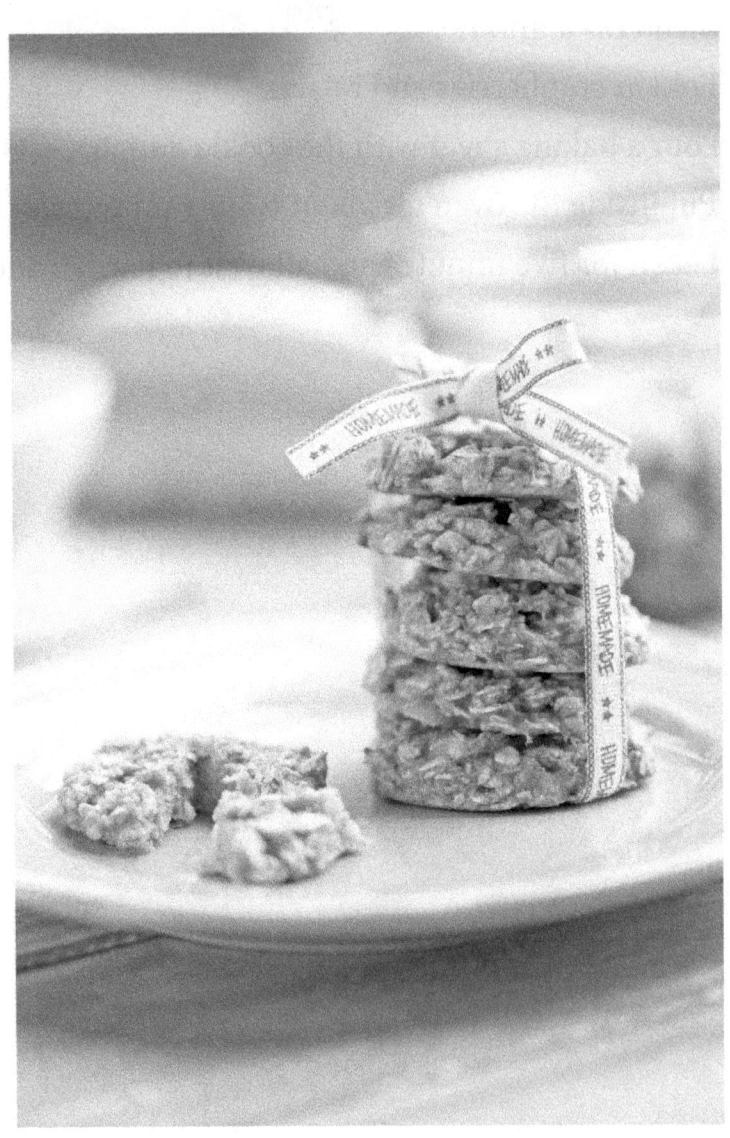

Berry Ice Pops

Time To Prepare: 3 Hours 5 Minutes
Time to Cook: 0 minutes
Yield: Servings 4

Ingredients:
- ¼ Cup Water
- 1 Cup Blueberries, Fresh or Frozen
- 1 Cup Strawberries, Fresh or Frozen
- 1 Teaspoon Lemon Juice, Fresh
- 2 Cups Whole Milk Yogurt, Plain
- 2 Tablespoons Honey, Raw

Directions:
1. Put all together the ingredients in a blender, and blend until the desired smoothness is achieved.
2. Pour into your molds, and freeze for minimum three hours before you serve

Berry-Banana Yogurt

Time To Prepare: ten minutes
Time to Cook: 0 minute
Yield: Servings 1

Ingredients:
- ¼ cup collard greens, chopped
- ¼ cup quick-cooking oats
- ½ banana, frozen fresh
- ½ cup blueberries, fresh and frozen
- 1 container 5.3 ounces Greek yogurt, non-fat
- 1 cup almond milk
- 5-6 ice cubes

Directions:
1. Take a microwave-safe cup and put in 1 cup almond milk and ¼ cup oats.
2. Put the cups into your microwave on high for 2.5 minutes.
3. When oats are cooked and 2 ice cubes to cool.
4. Combine them well.
5. Put in all ingredients in your blender Blend until smooth and creamy.
6. Best enjoyed chilled.

Blueberry Crisp

Time To Prepare: five minutes

Time to Cook: thirty minutes

Yield: Servings 4

Ingredients:
- ¼ cups pecans, chopped
- ¼ teaspoon nutmeg
- ½ teaspoon ginger
- 1 cup buckwheat
- 1 lb. blueberries
- 1 teaspoon of cinnamon
- 1 teaspoon of honey
- 2 tablespoons olive oil

Directions:
1. Preheat the oven to 350 degrees F.
2. Grease a baking dish.
3. Mix together the pecans, wheat, oil, spices, and honey in a container.
4. Put the berries in your pan.
5. Layer the topping on your berries.
6. Bake for thirty minutes at 350 F.

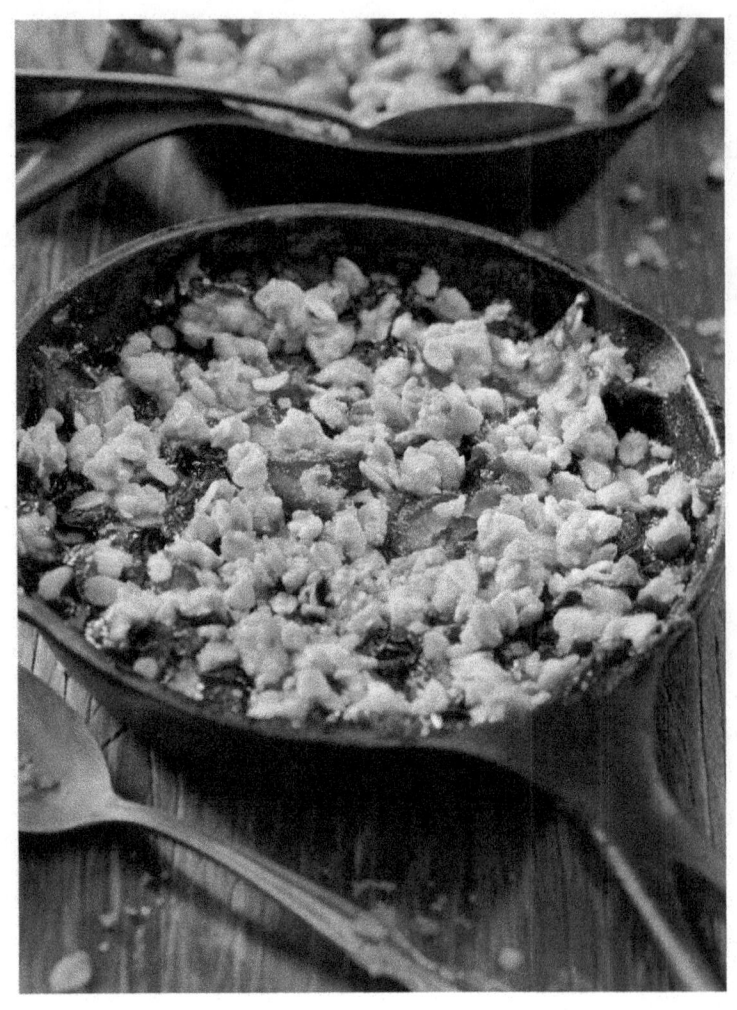

Blueberry Sour Cream Cake

Time To Prepare: twenty minutes

Time to Cook: 70 minutes

Yield: Servings 4

Ingredients:
- 1 Cup Blueberry
- 1 Cup Of Melted Butter
- 1 Cup Sour Cream
- 1 Tsp Vanilla Extract
- 1 Tsp. Baking Powder
- 1 Tsp. Cinnamon Powder
- 2 Cups Of Brown Sugar
- 2 Large Eggs
- 2 Tbsp. All-Purpose Flour Salt

Direction:

1. Preheat oven to 175C.
2. Mix together the butter and sugar till light and fluffy.
3. Put sour cream, vanilla extract, and eggs into the mixture.
4. In another container, put all together the dry ingredients then mix.

5. Place the dry mixture into the butter mixture, putting in blueberries, then mix well.

6. Put the batter into a greased pan then bake for about fifty minutes at 170C.

7. Serve with sour cream and blueberries.

Café-Style Fudge

Time To Prepare: ten minutes + chilling time

Time to Cook: 0 minutes

Yield: Servings 6

Ingredients:

- ½ teaspoon vanilla extract
- 1 stick butter
- 1 tablespoon instant coffee granules
- 4 tablespoons cocoa powder
- 4 tablespoons confectioners' Swerve

Directions:

1. Beat the butter and Swerve at low speed.

2. Put in the cocoa powder, instant coffee granules, and vanilla and continue to stir until well blended.

3. Ladle the batter into a foil-lined baking sheet.

4. Place in your fridge for two to three hours. Enjoy!

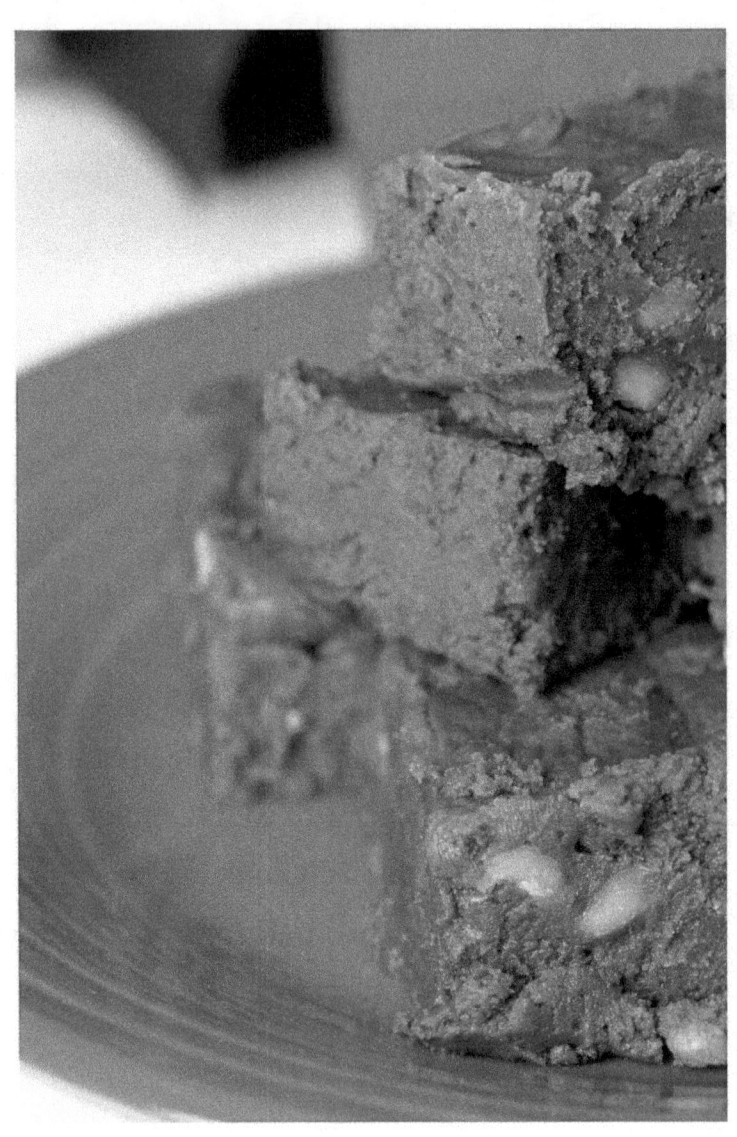

Grams Choco Chia Cherry Cream

Time To Prepare: 4 hours and five minutes
Time to Cook: 0 minutes
Yield: Servings 4

Ingredients:
- ¼-cup chia seeds, powdered
- ½-cup cherries, pitted and cut + extra for plating
- 1½-cups almond milk
- 2-Tbsps pure maple syrup or honey
- 3-Tbsps raw cacao, powdered

Additional toppings:
- extra raw cacao nibs, cherries, and 70% or higher dark chocolate shavings

Directions:
1. Mix in all the ingredients, excluding the cherries in a mason jar.
2. Mix thoroughly until meticulously blended.
3. Place in your fridge overnight or for 4 hours.
4. Before you serve, split the pudding equally among four serving plates.
5. Top each plate with the cherries.
6. Decorate using the additional toppings.

Chocolate Cherry Chia Pudding

Time To Prepare: 4 hours and five minutes

Time to Cook: 0 minutes

Yield: Servings 4

Ingredients:
- ¼ cup Chia seeds You can also use chia seed powder.
- ½ cup Sliced pitted cherries
- 1 ½ cup Any non-dairy milk like coconut or almond milk
- 3 tbsp. Maple syrup or honey
- 3 tbsp. Raw cacao powder

Additional toppings:
- Dark chocolate shavings (Preferably 70% dark chocolate or more)
- Extra cherries
- Raw cacao nibs

Directions:
1. Use a mason jar or a container.
2. If you're using a container, just pour in the milk, maple syrup, chia seeds or powder, and raw cacao.

3. Stir meticulously and place in your fridge for 4 hours or more.

4. If you decide to use a mason jar, just pour in the same ingredients, screw the lid on and shake vigorously!

5. Serve in separate dishes and top with any or all of the toppings I listed above.

6. Enjoy!

Chocolate Chip Quinoa Granola Bars

Time To Prepare: five minutes

Time to Cook: ten minutes

Yield: Servings 16

Ingredients:
- ¼ teaspoon salt
- ½ cup flax seed
- ½ cup of chia seeds
- ½ cup of chocolate chips
- ½ cup of honey
- ½ cup walnuts, chopped
- 1 cup buckwheat
- 1 cup uncooked quinoa
- 1 teaspoon of cinnamon
- 1 teaspoon of vanilla
- 2/3 cup dairy-free margarine

Directions:
1. Preheat the oven to 350 degrees F.
2. Spread the walnuts, quinoa, wheat, flax, and chia on your baking sheet.
3. Bake for about ten minutes.

4. Coat a baking dish using plastic wrap. Line with cooking spray. Keep aside.

5. Melt the margarine and honey in a saucepot.

6. Mix together the vanilla, salt, and cinnamon into the margarine mix.

7. Keep the wheat mix and quinoa in a container.

8. Pour the margarine sauce into it. Mix the mixture. Coat well. Let it cool. Mix in the chocolate chips.

9. Spread your mixture into the baking dish.

10. Push tightly into the pan. Plastic wrap.

11. Place in your fridge overnight.

12. Cut into bars and serve.

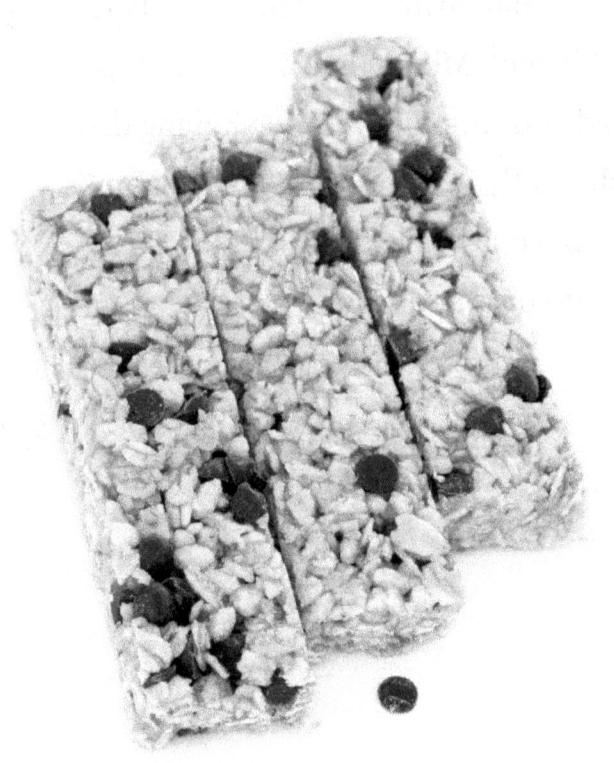

Chocolate Fudge Bites

TimeTo Prepare: ten minutes

Time to Cook: three minutes

Yield: Servings 10

Ingredients:

- ½ cup of coconut milk powder
- ½ cup of cold water
- ½ cup of raw cocoa powder
- 1 and a ¼ cup of boiling water
- 1 cup of coconut oil
- 1/3 cup of pure maple syrup 3 tablespoons of grass-fed gelatin

Directions:

1. Mix one and a quarter cup of boiling water with the gelatin, and boil for about three minutes.
2. Next, put the gelatin mixture into a blender with the cold water and rest of the ingredients.
3. Blend for about 2 minutes to help the gelatin solidify.
4. Put the mixture into the bottom of a greased baking dish, then place in your fridge until firm.
5. Cut into little serving squares.

Cinnamon Apple Chips

Time To Prepare: 10 Minutes

Time to Cook: 2 Hours

Yield: Servings 3

Ingredients:
- ¾ tsp. Cinnamon, grounded
- 3 Honey crisp Apple, big & sweet

Directions:

1. For making this dessert fare, preheat your oven to 200 ° F.
2. Next, keep a parchment paper-lined baking sheet in the center and lower rack.
3. With the help of an apple corer, core the apples and then slice the apples into 1/8-inch-thick rounds.
4. Next, position the apples in the preheated baking sheet in a single layer.
5. After this, drizzle the cinnamon over the apples.
6. Once sprinkled, bake them for an hour.
7. Take away the baking sheet and then switch their position.
8. Bake them for another one to 1 ½ hour or until the chips are crunchy.

9. To finish, once they are crisp in accordance with your liking, remove the apple chips from the oven.

10. Let the chips cool for one hour before you serve.

Citrus Strawberry Granita

Time To Prepare: fifteen minutes
Time to Cook: 0 minutes
Yield: Servings 4

Ingredients:
- ¼ cup of raw honey
- ¼ lemon
- 1 grapefruit (peeled, seeded, and sectioned)
- 12 ounces of fresh strawberries, hulled
- 2 oranges (peeled, seeded and sectioned)

Directions:
1. Put strawberries, grapefruit, oranges, and lemon in a juicer and extract juice according to the manufacturer's instructions.
2. Put 1½ cups of the veggie juice and honey to a pan and cook on moderate heat for five minutes while stirring constantly.
3. Remove it from heat and put it in the rest of the juice.
4. Set aside for roughly thirty minutes.
5. Move the juice mixture into an 8x8-inch glass baking dish.
6. Freeze for 4 hours while scraping after every thirty minutes

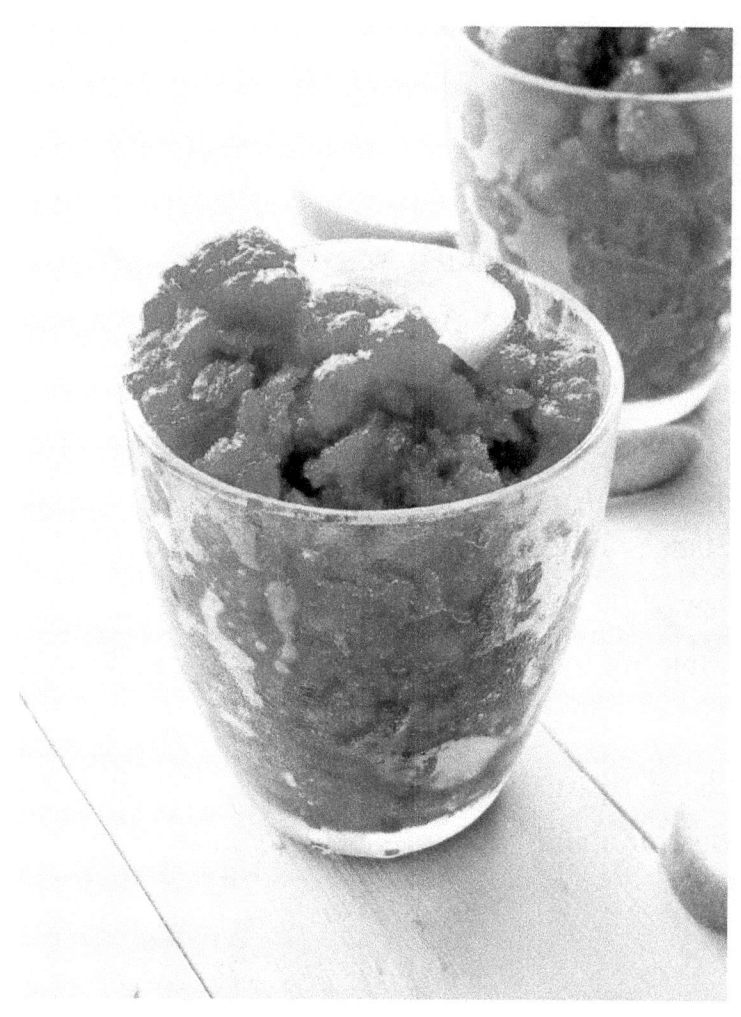

Coconut Butter Fudge

Time To Prepare: ten minutes

Time to Cook: 0 minutes

Yield: Servings 6

Ingredients:
- ¼ teaspoon of salt
- 1 cup of coconut butter
- 1 teaspoon of pure vanilla extract
- 2 tablespoons of raw honey

Directions:

1. Start by lining an 8 x 8 inch baking dish using parchment paper.
2. Melt the coconut butter, honey, and vanilla using low heat.
3. Place the mixture into the baking pan, and place in your fridge for about two hours before you serve.

Coffee Cream

TimeTo Prepare: ten minutes

Time to Cook: fifteen minutes

Yield: Servings 4

Ingredients:
- ¼ cup brewed coffee
- 1 teaspoon vanilla extract
- 2 cups heavy cream
- 2 eggs
- 2 tablespoons ghee, melted
- 2 tablespoons swerve

Directions:

1. In a container, mix the coffee with the cream and the other ingredients, whisk well and split it into 4 ramekins and whisk well.

2. Introduce the ramekins in your oven at 350 degrees F and bake for fifteen minutes.

3. Serve warm

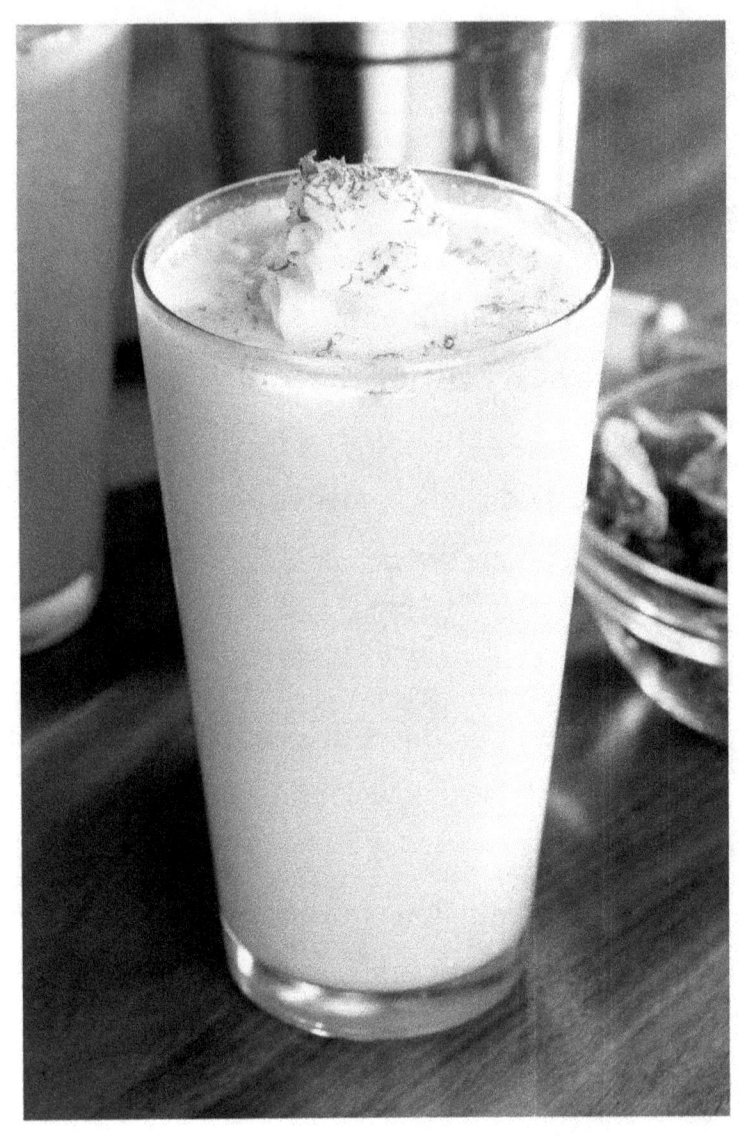

Cookie Dough Bites

Time To Prepare: 10 Minutes
Time to Cook: 5 Minutes
Yield: Servings 2

Ingredients:
- ¼ cup Almond Flour
- ¼ cup Chocolate Chips, dairy-free & sugar-free
- ½ cup Almond Butter or any nut butter
- ½ tsp. Salt
- 1 ½ cups Chickpeas, cooked
- 1 tsp. Vanilla Extract
- 2 tbsp. Maple Syrup

Directions:
1. First, place all the ingredients excluding the chocolate chips in a high-speed blender for about three minutes or until you get a thick, smooth mixture.
2. After this, move the mixture to a moderate-sized container.
3. Next, fold in the chocolate chips into the batter.
4. Check for sweetness and put in more maple syrup if required.
5. Serve and enjoy.

Creamy Frozen Yogurt

Time To Prepare: ten minutes + 2-three hours freezing

Time to Cook:

Yield: Servings 3

Ingredients:
- ½ cup of coconut yogurt
- ½ cup of unsweetened almond milk
- 1 tbsp. of raw honey
- 1 tsp. of fresh mint leaves
- 1 tsp. of organic vanilla extract
- 2 peeled, pitted and chopped medium avocados
- 2 tbsp. of fresh lemon juice

Directions:
1. Throw all the ingredients into a blender apart from mint leaves and pulse till creamy and smooth.
2. Put into an airtight container then freeze for minimum 2- three hours.
3. Take off from the freezer and keep aside for about fifteen minutes. With a spoon stir thoroughly.
4. Top with fresh mint leaves before you serve.

Date Dough & Walnut Wafer

Time To Prepare: fifteen minutes

Time to Cook: eighteen minutes

Yield: Servings 8

Ingredients:
- ¼-cup coconut oil
- ¼-tsp sea salt
- ½-cup coconut, unsweetened
- ½-cup walnuts
- ½-tsp baking soda
- ½-tsp sea salt
- 1½-cup oats (divided)
- 18-pcs Medjool dates, pitted
- 1-pc egg
- 1-tsp lemon juice
- 2-Tbsps ground flaxseed
- 6-pcs Medjool dates, pitted and cut into four equivalent portions

For the Date Layer:

Directions:

1. Preheat the oven to 325°F.

2. Coat a baking pan using parchment paper.

3. Pulse a cup of oats in a food processor until making a flour consistency.

4. Put in the dates, coconut, baking soda, and sea salt.

5. Pulse again until the dates completely break up.

6. Put in the remaining oats and walnuts, and pulse until the nuts break, but still a bit lumpy. Put in the flaxseed, egg, and oil.

7. Pulse the mixture further until meticulously blended.

8. Set aside ½-cup of the date mixture to use as a topping later.

9. Push down the rest of the mix to a uniform layer in the pan.

10. Wash your food processor, and put in all the date layer ingredients.

11. Pulse the mixture until the dates completely break up and take on a light caramel color.

12. With wet hands, press the mixture down, smoothing it on the date mixture.

13. Crumble and drizzle the reserved date mixture over the top.

14. Place the pan in your oven. Bake for eighteen minutes.

15. Allow the wafer to cool to room temperature before cutting into 16 pieces.

Fall-Time Custard

Time To Prepare: fifteen minutes
Time to Cook: 60 minutes
Yield: Servings 6

Ingredients:
- ¼ tsp. of ground ginger
- 1 cup of canned pumpkin
- 1 cup of coconut milk
- 1 tsp. of ground cinnamon
- 1 tsp. of organic vanilla extract
- 2 organic eggs
- 2 pinches of freshly grated nutmeg
- 8-10 drops of liquid stevia
- Pinch of salt

Directions:
1. Preheat your oven to 350 degrees F.
2. In a big container, put together pumpkin and spices then mix.
3. In another container, put in the eggs and beat thoroughly.
4. Put in the rest of the ingredients then whisk till well blended.

5. Put in egg mixture into pumpkin mixture and mix till well blended.

6. Move the mixture to 6 ramekins.

7. Position the ramekins in a baking dish, Put in sufficient water in the baking dish about two-inch high around the ramekins.

8. Bake for approximately 1 hour or till a toothpick inserted in the middle comes out clean

Flourless Sweet Potato Brownies

Time To Prepare: ten minutes

Time to Cook: thirty minutes

Yield: Servings 9

Ingredients:

- ¼ cup Unsweetened Cocoa powder
- ½ cup Almond butter
- ½ cup Cooked sweet potato
- ½ tsp. Baking soda
- 1 big Whole egg
- 2 tsp. Vanilla extract
- 3 tbsp. Dairy-free chocolate chips, optional.
- 6 tbsp. Honey

Directions:

1. Prep the oven by preheating to 350°F.
2. Coat a baking pan using parchment paper leaving a few extra inches on the sides to make it easier to discard or remove
3. Blend all the ingredients, excluding the chocolate chips until you get a super smooth and tender batter.
4. Move the creamy batter to your readied baking pan and use a spatula to spread it around, so it looks almost even.

5. Slide it in your oven, then bake for thirty minutes or until a knife inserted into the pan comes out clean.

6. Remove from the oven and leave to cool in the pan for fifteen minutes before putting it up on a wire rack.

7. If you decide to use the chocolate chip topping, put the chips in a microwave-safe dish and heat until it completely melts.

8. Remove from the microwave and sprinkle over the brownies.

9. Serve or store!

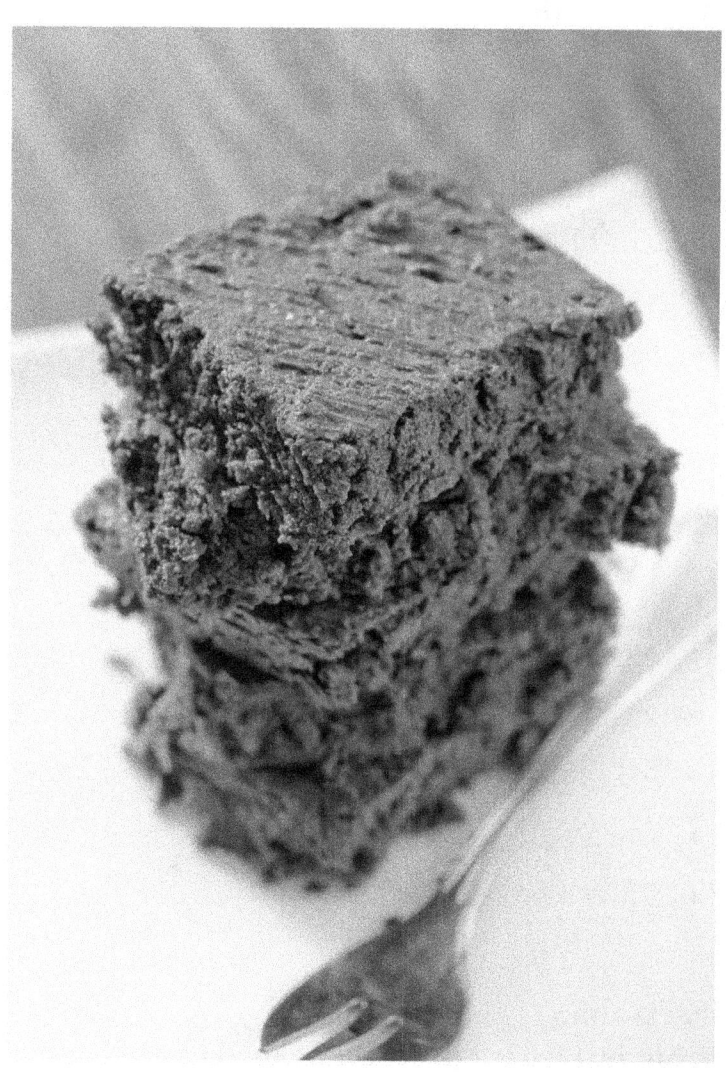

Fruit Cobbler

Time To Prepare: ten minutes
Time to Cook: twenty minutes
Yield: Servings 8

Ingredients:
- ¼ Cup Coconut Oil, Melted
- ¼ Cup Coconut Sugar
- ½ Teaspoon Vanilla Extract, Pure
- ¾ Cup Almond Flour
- ¾ Cup Rolled Oats
- 1 Teaspoon Coconut Oil
- 1 Teaspoon Ground Cinnamon
- 2 Cups Nectarines, Fresh & Sliced
- 2 Cups Peaches, Fresh & Sliced
- 2 Tablespoons Lemon Juice, Fresh
- Dash Salt
- Filter Water for Mixing

Directions:
1. Begin by heating the oven to 425.
2. Get out a cast-iron frying pan, coating it with a teaspoon of coconut oil.

3. Mix your lemon juice, peaches, and nectarines together in the frying pan.

4. Prepare your food processor, mixing your almond flour, oats, coconut sugar, and remaining coconut oil.

5. Put in your cinnamon, vanilla, and salt, pulsing until the oat mixture looks like a dry dough. If you need more moisture, put in filtered water a tablespoon at a time, and then break the dough into chunks, spreading it across the fruit.

6. Bake for 20 minutes before you serve warm.

Glazed Banana

Time To Prepare: ten minutes
Time to Cook: five minutes
Yield: Servings 2

Ingredients:
- 1 peeled and cut under-ripened banana
- 1 tbsp. of filtered water
- 1 tbsp. of olive oil
- 1 tbsp. of raw honey
- 1/8 tsp. of ground cinnamon

Directions:
1. In a nonstick frying pan, warm oil on moderate heat.
2. Put in banana slices and cook for approximately 1-2 minutes per side.
3. In the meantime, in a small container, put in water and honey and beat thoroughly.
4. Move the banana slices on a serving plate. Instantly, pour honey mixture over banana slices.
5. Keep aside to cool to room temperature.
6. Serve with the drizzling of cinnamon

Green Tea Pudding

Time To Prepare: twenty minutes

Time to Cook: ten minutes

Yield: Servings 3

Ingredients:
- 1 Tsp. Matcha Green Tea Powder
- 1/4 Cup Brown Sugar
- 1/4 Cup Corn Starch
- 1/8-Tbsp. Cinnamon Powder
- 100g Butter
- 2 Cup Heavy Milk
- 3 Eggs Salt

Directions:

1. In a big pot, mix brown sugar, milk, cornstarch, and matcha powder.
2. In moderate heat, keep whisking until combined.
3. Combine the hot batter with whisked eggs slowly.
4. Cook for three to five minutes.
5. Strain the mixture and put in butter.
6. Place the mixture in a container, place in your fridge for a few hours before you serve.

Hot Chocolate

Time To Prepare: 5 Minutes
Time to Cook: 5 Minutes
Yield: Servings 2

Ingredients:
- ¼ tsp. Turmeric
- ½ tsp. Cinnamon
- 1 tbsp. Coconut Oil
- 1 tbsp. Honey, raw
- 2 cups Almond Milk
- 2 tbsp. Cocoa Powder, unsweetened

Directions:
1. To start with, bring the almond milk to its boiling point in a deep deep cooking pan on moderate heat.
2. Now, bring this mixture to a simmer and then mix in the cocoa powder to it.
3. Next, spoon in the turmeric powder and cinnamon to it. Mix thoroughly
4. Next, put in honey to it and once blended well, put in the coconut oil.
5. Give the drink a good stir until everything comes together.
6. Serve instantly.

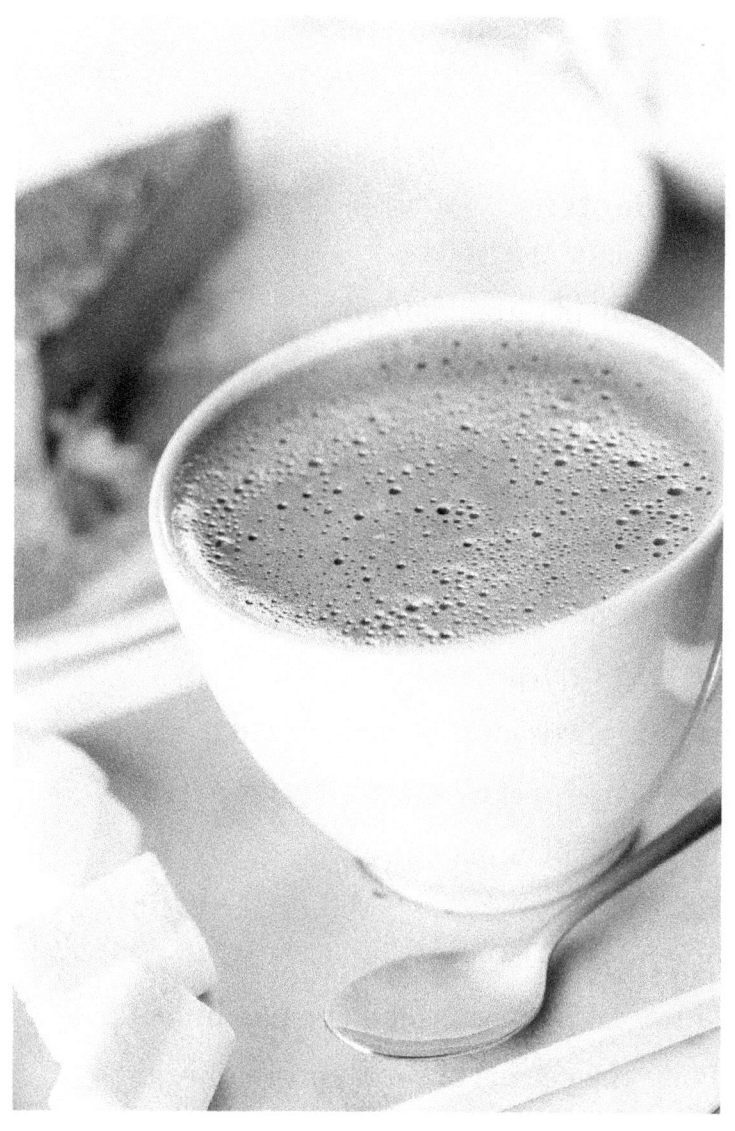

Lemon Vegan Cake

Time To Prepare: ten minutes

Time to Cook: ten minutes

Yield: Servings 3

Ingredients:
- ½ lemon extract
- 1 cup of pitted dates
- 1 lemon juice and zest
- 1½ cup agave
- 1½ cups of dairy-free yogurt
- 1½ cups pineapple, crushed
- 1½ teaspoon vanilla extract
- 2½ cups pecans
- ½ 3 avocados, halved & pitted
- 3 cups of cauliflower rice, prepared
- Pinch of cinnamon

Directions:
1. Line your baking sheet using parchment paper.
2. Pulse the pecans in a food processor.
3. Put in the agave and dates.
4. Pulse for one minute.

5. Move this mix to the baking sheet. Wipe the container of your processor.

6. Combine the pineapple, agave, avocados, cauliflower, lemon juice, and zest in a food processor.

7. Pulse till smooth Now put in the lemon extract, cinnamon, and vanilla extract. Pulse.

8. Pour this mix into your pan, on the crust.

9. Place in your fridge for around five hours at least.

10. Take out the cake and keep it at room temperature for about twenty minutes.

11. Take out the cake's outer ring.

12. Mix together the vanilla extract, agave, and yogurt in a container.

13. Pour on your cake

Notes

www.ingramcontent.com/pod-product-compliance
Lightning Source LLC
Chambersburg PA
CBHW070723030426
42336CB00013B/1902